Disclaimer

This book is a work of the author's experiences and opinions. Names, characters, places, and incidents are the product of the author's imagination. In no way, shape, or form is this diet book connected with the Fear Factor TV series or any parts there of.

ISBN-13 978-1475077117
Cover design by Greg Ryan
Email: greg@resolutions.bz
website: www.resolutions.bz
Blogs: www.resolutionsblog.com
www.gregryanfitness.com

Why you should read this book?

These may be the only words you will hear that are sincere and to the point. The *"Fear" Factor* is written not for you to feel fluffy inside, but to force you to see the reality, or I should say, illusion, that you have created in your head which is preventing you from losing weight.

This book does not mince words and may come across much more straight forward than you would like. I cannot help you there. We do not always like what we hear, but at the same time we NEED to hear it. These words could just very well save our lives some day.

Losing weight is not complicated people, but acknowledging why you are not may be. You need to read this book to convince yourself you deserve to feel better, even if it is just for one day! Losing weight comes down to one word!

About the Author

Greg Ryan's career began thirty years ago, at age 45, as a professional fitness trainer. In 1986 he won his first of two Michigan bodybuilding championships.

He won his second title in 1988. In 1990, he moved to Los Angeles California, where his knowledge, enthusiasm, and skill attracted the attention of fitness guru Kathy Smith.

During this time, Greg ran one of the largest personal training businesses in LA. This attracted numerous high profile movies stars such as Brooke Shields, Bridget Fonda, Connie Sellecca, and many more. Greg built a reputation for exercise and behavior change and in the fall of 1992 appeared on the Today Show and Good Morning America.

In 1994, Greg returned to college to further his knowledge in Physical Therapy. During this time Greg's gift of motivating individuals led him to the production of his own television segment on FOX TV.

In 1997 Greg relocated to Louisville, Kentucky were he built and operated a private clinic specializing in obesity and diabetic weight loss programs. Numerous bodybuilding titles, movie star clients, and over a dozen authored books and counting has made him one of the most experienced and sought after experts in the business. Today, Greg has acquired almost one hundred thousand hours of personal training to go with his well rounded career.

From the Author

Individuals do not have an educational problem when it comes to losing weight. It is a motivational one. Deep down, you know what you should do and what you should not, but do you do it? No. So there lies the issue. The so called experts and doctors say we just need to educate, which is bull crap. I beg to differ, we need to motivate and that sometimes requires going against political correctness.

I am the Simon Cowell of fitness, not a psychologist, but I have learned a few things over the years. I do not mince words and straight talk is what you will get. I am writing this book to save lives, not to make friends. You are over weight for a reason and first you must acknowledge the WHY's behind the reason. The sad thing is, most, if not all, the hang ups you have, you have created in your mind and they are false, whether you admit them or not. The biggest challenge you will have reading this book is controlling your anger, not with me, but with yourself. Get over it!

If you want a quick fix to your weight problem then stop reading right now and go buy a late night info commercial gadget, but if you TRULY want to figure things out, open up your mind and read on…..

Content

Introduction

Part 1: Face to Face- (Facing the Problem)

1. Face to Face
2. Keeping It Simple
3. The Root of It All
4. The Silent Killers
5. Avoid the ER – Exercise Resistance (of the mind)

Part 2: AAA Coverage- (Solving the Problem)

6. Acceptance
7. Attitudes
8. Attractions

Part 3: Action Cures Frustration

9. Just Move It

Part 4: Food for Thought (thoughts on food)

10. Planning for Weight Loss
11. Five P's for Guaranteed Weight Reduction
12. Red Flags

Part 5: Just One (the mind set)

13. Just One

Part 6: The "Fear" Factor- (the Illusion)

14. The Fear Factor

Bonus Material

Ten Commandments to Lowering Your Body-Fat!

The reason you are not losing weight comes down to one word, like it or not! That word is fueled by two other words and they control the other three words that keep you from losing weight.

Greg Ryan

Introduction

It has been almost thirty years since that first day I stepped foot in that old run down health club in the basement of the guys dormitory at Andrews University. I wonder what the two of them were thinking. I never asked, but I could only imagine. Scared would not be the word I would use to describe how I felt as I stood there, right in the middle of the workout floor. I was frozen stiff with fear of what I was about to get myself into. The problem was, I had absolutely no clue what to do or what was about to happen.

Fitness found me at the lowest point in my life. I did not realize it at the time, but looking back it was a scary time. *Fear* ran through my veins like syrup and fat hung on my body like meat in a super market. I had a personality like a box of rocks and a self confidence level that amounted to little, if anything, and was made for a bad movie.

Then, one day, I had a little talk with my self and they all left; the voices that is. The sounds in my head of resentment; failure; high expectations; comparisons; envy; jealousy; pride; denial; and even a bit of laziness all left. Just like that? Just like that.

It is amazing what a dose of reality, common sense, and one simple question will do for a life. For me, it changed it for ever and ever.

Do I still have tough days? You bet. Do I still have voices in my head at times? Absolutely I do. The difference now is that I know what to do in order to get over the hang ups.

Losing weight is not as challenging physically as it is mentally, at least long term that is. *"Guard your Hearts and Minds,"* the good book says. It is really true as it pertains to your weight loss success. Your biggest competitor is you. You have no one else to blame for the lack of accountability, but on the flip side you can take all the credit for your successes.

Part 1
Face to Face
(Facing the Problem)

1
Face to Face

We live in a world now that promotes taking the road less traveled, being politically correct, and if it has any aspect of common sense, it must not be right.

Our weight problem in America is just a microcosm of the overall issue our country is facing. We are taught to push the negative circumstances down the road in hopes that we will never have to face them. An *"Out of sight, out of mind,"* type of thinking. Take a look at Diabetes for a moment. You cannot see Diabetes because it is an internal disease. If we cannot see it, then we take no serious interest in preventing it. Then when the doctor diagnoses you with it, you act shocked and mad.

Pay Now or Pay Later

Why have I allowed myself to get into this kind of shape?

With life comes responsibility and with decisions comes consequences.

Sooner or later you will be in front of the piper and you can pay him now or you can pay later. If you wait, interest will accrue in the form of pain and/or inconvenience. There is no getting around that. Just look at our economy, the payment has come due, plus interest.

Look at the housing market, car industry, or AIG insurance. Financial planners teach people to have an emergency fund for just that, an emergency. If you do not have such a fund, you will pay a bigger price when you need money for a crisis. My point is; let us face the facts now, on our own terms, rather than sometime soon down the road.

Losing weight today, despite what you think, is not that complicated. Sure, it takes discipline, but the path to get there is pretty much straight as an arrow. The problem is people value things that more costly or complicated. If it is simple, it must not work. If there is no drama, it will be boring.

The reason you are not losing weight comes down to one word, like it or not! That word is fueled by two others and they control the other three words that keep you from dropping the pounds.

2
Keeping It Simple

K.I.S.S... This may come of a shock to you, but losing weight is not that complicated. Yet, most people want to think that it is. For some reason, if it seems confusing, hard to follow, or complicated, then it must work. Wrong!

Keep the Process Simple

People want to make losing weight complicated and/or difficult, and then, when they fail, they can blame their failure on the complexity of it all. If it were easy, then there would be no excuses for the failure. Guess what? It is easier than you think and your failure to follow through is only an excuse.

Common Sense

There are NO magic formulas or equipment to help you lose weight, SORRY! So what is missing in people's fitness programs? In short, one thing is common sense. Yes, common sense. Most think if a book has any value, it must be written by a book scholar or professor in order to be true. This is simply not true.

Most individuals believe you have to be a math genius to calculate calories and weight loss graphs. This is not true either. In the process, all of these books and diet programs are being promoted and you are getting fatter. What most do not notice is each sales pitch is missing a common ingredient, COMMON SENSE.

Losing weight has more to do with common sense than any other ingredient in your diet plan. The problem is common sense is FREE and anything free in the world is usually looked over, frowned upon, and/or deemed worthless.

Bite Sizes

Losing weight is also about bite sizes, not just eating wise, but it is a mental challenge as well.

The New Years Resolution Problem

Today, as a matter of fact, is New Year's Day. The attitude of people today, who want to lose weight, is much different than those in the past. In my book, **"Why Wait,"** I explain the main reason people fail to keep New Year's Fitness Resolutions. This is because they bite off more than they can chew. Trying to go from not exercising at all to working out five days a week is impossible for the mind to comprehend.

Well, that is exactly what you are trying to do when you make New Year's fitness resolutions.

If you learn nothing else from this book, remember these two things; fear and bite sizes.

F.E.A.R.

False- Evidence- Appearing- Real

3
The Root of It All

I truly believe at the core, the number one reason people do not lose weight comes down to a single emotion. While diet and exercise are a must, this one emotion can single handedly destroy a person INSIDE OUT. Without a doubt, the most powerful force on earth, when it comes to motivating people to do or not do something, lies in these four letters; F.E.A.R..

Nature Born Killers

Do you know there are only two naturally born fears? The first is fear of falling and the second is loud noises. All the other fears people have are learned behavior, so that means they can be unlearned, right?

No matter how you slice it, *fear* is the root of it all. As crazy as it may sound, you are not losing weight because you are fearful. Maybe not directly or consciences, but fear fuels so many other powerful emotions. Fortunately, your fears are not real.

Delusions

Delusions are false beliefs that we have created in our minds. They are always pathological, despite over whelming evidence against it. If you have delusions, are you a mental case? This is absolutely not true. The mind can and will play games with you.

Your mind will twist the actual truth of a situation. In this book we will discuss three feelings in later chapters that go along with FEAR and weight loss.

Just keep in mind, most, if not all, of the things that keep you from starting or following through on a fitness plan to lose weight are FALSE. There is an acronym we use for the word FEAR.

False-Evidence-Appearing-Real

False

When something is false, it means that there are no facts to back up the statement. All of your thoughts concerning why, how, when, and where you cannot lose weight are UN truths.

You may think these things are true, but at their core, they are not. There is no evidence to back up your mind's claims. The sad thing is you have made them your reality.

Evidence

Evidence is the facts of a given situation. What evidence do you have proving that you do not deserve to lose weight or be healthier?

Appearing

Appearing is things that you see, or perhaps more accurately, think you see. In other words, it is what you *believe* you are seeing. You can convince yourself into believing it is the truth when it is not.

Real

Real is things that physically exist and are not imaginary. You have actual facts to back it up with.

Over view

When it comes to your weight loss problems, the first thing to do is establish the root of why you do not lose weight or fail to follow through on an exercise program.

We have done that; FEAR. You may not admit it, but most likely you are scared or *think* you are frightened. We have established that all that all emotion is totally FALSE, no matter how you slice it! You or someone else has fed that to your brain and over time you have come to believe it.

K.I.S.S.

4
The Silent Killers

Now that we have established the root of your weight loss problem, we still have not solved the issue. There are feelings that go with a strong core emotion. This is where it gets interesting. While the number one reason people do not lose weight is *fear,* there are three feelings that motivate each individual to do or not do things. One, or all, can single handedly bring you down and possibly kill you.

The key to your weight loss success lies in overcoming three feelings that are rooted in fear: *denial, pride and laziness.* It is safe to say, **Denial** may be the strongest of the three because it is so far under the radar, rooted deep in the mind.

The Silent Killer

Has denial ever made you think things like, *"My diet is not that bad."*? How about,*"A few trips to the fast food joint once in a while will not hurt."*

Have you ever said to yourself, "My blood pressure is fine; it will not hurt if I skip a day of taking my medication"?

"My New Year's resolution is to get in better shape."

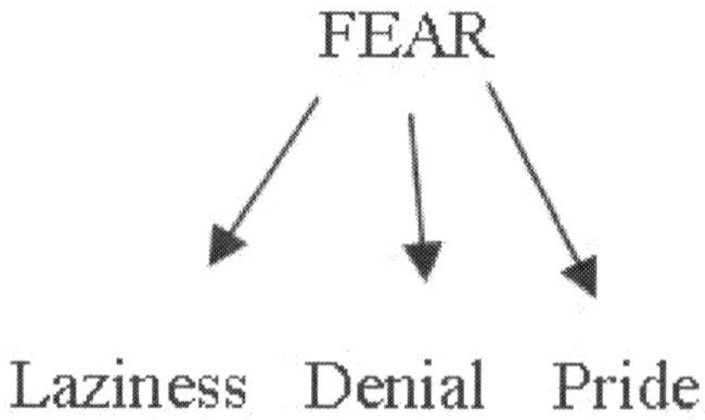
FEAR
Laziness
Denial
Pride

"Whyhave I let myself get this out of shape?

Or "It will not happen to me…no way!"

Unfortunately, it is what is not seen that is killing you. Your insides are being eaten up ever so slowly, both physically and emotionally. Physically your health is suffering because of lack of activity and poor eating habits. Emotionally, your self-esteem suffers because you are not facing the facts, leading to a slow and painful death of the soul and possibly a physical one in the end.

Society is so concerned with makeover television shows that we have been caught off guard by silent killers, such as heart disease, diabetes, and obesity. We overlook the long-term consequence of our behavior. We see things going on around us, but we continue to put off exercise and eating better for another day.

Denying something is a lot easier in the beginning, but sooner or later the truth with come calling.

Dealing with life on your terms is so much better than having to react to life on its own pay ground. Pay now or pay later! *Denial is followed by pride!*

Pride goeth before the fall

Ever find yourself saying or thinking, *"If I cannot do it on my own, then I will not do it at all."*

"Just the very fact of having to take better care of myself, irritates me."

"I'll put off my check up until next fall."

First, let me say there are two different ways of looking at pride; taking pride or stubborn pride. My father would say,

"Son never let them see you sweat or they may think you are weak."

Other times, he would encourage me to, *"Take Pride"* in my work. In other words, care. Both perspectives are forms of pride; one is a positive and up lifting, while the other is ego and low self esteem.

Pride fuels the engine of denial, which runs the car of laziness!

Greg Ryan

The positive side of pride is when you *"take pride"* in something and when you feel good about a project, event, or objective. The negative side of pride reveals feelings of stubbornness, envy, and even resentment. I believe pride costs thousands of lives every year by encouraging inactivity and depression.

Why be so stubborn? It is your health so why care what others feel? Why is your ego so strong that it is so paralyzing that you do not do anything? If you think about it, this way of thinking is really down right stupid.

Lazy is what lazy does

"I'll start tomorrow on an exercise program."

Exercise and eating healthy takes discipline and for some that is too much to ask. If that is you, then you may be missing out on a really wonderful, healthy, and quality filled life. Perhaps that is not even enough motivation for you.

Why is America the fattest nation in the world? Pure laziness! It is just that simple. If you think a pill, surgery, or wishful thinking is going to replace hard work, then you have been HAD by the media. It takes consistent work and even hard work at times.

Learned Helplessness

Learned helplessness is basically when someone or society does something for you that you are fully capable of doing it yourself. Over time, this behavior becomes a feeling of helplessness and even entitlement. Something that was meant for good can be turned into learned helplessness…e.g. the welfare system. It is not the fault of the system, but those who have taken advantage of it.

Technology

Rick Pitino, one of my favorite basketball coaches, said once,

"Technology is ruining our athletes; they are more concerned with pleasing their friends on "Face Book" and reading their text messages after a game rather than just playing the game for themselves or the love of it."

Email systems have disconnected people and genuine communication has suffered. Text messaging has almost dismantled the spelling and English system. People have become addicted to technology and the high that it gives them.

Recently, our town suffered an ice storm and my email was down for a week. I truly felt uncomfortable and out of whack. How sad is that?

I will not even get into the effects of video games.

Protectionism

Protectionism is a word that describes how kids and some adults are treated these days.

I grew up on a farm and rarely did I ever get sick. One of the neighbor boys always seemed to have a cold. We never understood why his mother would always make him dress in the summer like it was the dead of winter. Another neighbor boy, who is thirty- five years old now, still lives with his parents.

My nephew's school teacher is getting sued by the parents of another child for calling him out in front of the others; apparently he spit on one of his class mates. The parents felt their child's discipline was unwarranted and caused undue stress and embarrassment, so they filed a complaint against the teacher.

Kids these days get away with so much and are handed more than any of the previous generations.

If they fail or fall short of expectations, there is someone right there to make an excuse for them or put the blame on something else.

There is a shortage of accountability these days. While society thinks it is protecting people, the reality is the opposite. It is weakening the spirit and our survival instincts. The sad thing is that learned helplessness, laziness, pride, and denial are all have some sort of price to be paid.

DO NOT FORGET TO READ THE LAST CHAPTER!

5
Avoiding the ER!

Why is it so hard for me to start exercising? I know it is good for me. It seems like I have some form of resistance to getting in better shape.

"Exercise Resistance" or ***ER*** means a conscious or unconscious block against participating in a regular, active program. Studies show that some people have built up barriers because of past experiences that create a negative mindset about exercise and food. In many cases, this prevents a person from starting or following through on an exercise program.

We all have barriers that come in different forms of emotions. Each barrier is usually due to an experience we have had, someone telling us a bold face lie about ourselves in a particular situation, or we have made up some delusional thought on our own.

Resentment

I thought the golden years were supposed to be filled with relaxing things to do, not with more activities that I would usually put off before?

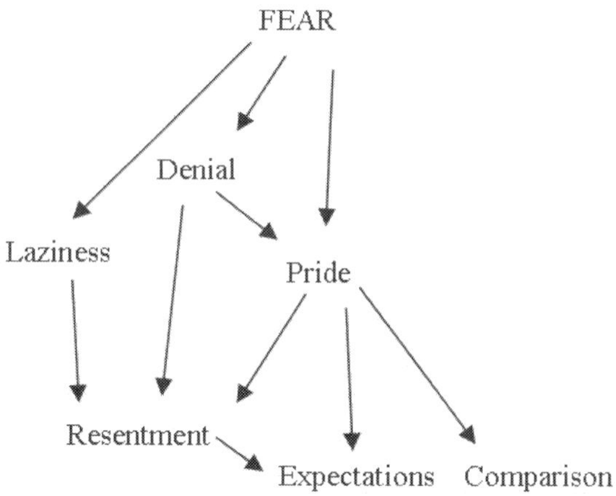
FEAR
Denial
Laziness
Pride
Resentment
Expectations
Comparison

I hate the way I look. In my twenty's I could get away with eating just about anything!

Not wanting to exercise is one thing, but resenting exercise can be paralyzing. Truly, there are only a small percentage of people who like to exercise. Many individuals do it for a sport or profession. Most people hate the effort, but they love the results.

Resentment toward exercise goes much deeper than just not liking the effort; it brings out rebellious attitudes. As we get older, we grow more frustrated and boundaries have to be set. We may even act like a little child at times. We stomp our feet, cross our arms, and pout thinking:

"You cannot tell me what to do; I will show you."

The sooner you accept the fact that exercise is going to be a part of your life, the more likely you are to start and the more likely you are to continue. Resentment is fueled by being in denial or full of pride.

Failure

Why should I start exercising? I will not follow through. I never have before. It will be just another failure.

The only failure is not starting. Success is not measured in numbers. It is measured in your growth through the process. Just because your track record may show some ups and downs has no bearing on your future efforts. Your self-worth is not based on how many times you started an exercise program.

I would rather try and feel good about my efforts, even if I did not succeed, rather than have the feeling of regret for never having tried. *Fear of failure is just an excuse to never try.*

Perfection

"Why am I not doing this the way I know how? I might as well not do it at all."

If you think for a second that you are going to be perfect sticking to a plan, then you might as well forget it. The truth is that it will never go the way you want it to. Life brings hurdles, road blocks, and forks in the road. If you are frightened about being perfect, then your intentions are not internal, but are for pleasing someone else.

Let me tell you a little secret, no one else really cares if you get a hundred or fail, they really only care about themselves. They will forget about you in a day no matter what the out come is. *Perfectionism is an illusion.*

Comparisons

Why do people like Jane look like they do and I have to work so hard? It does not seem fair!"

News flash; life is not fair! For some, it seems effortless to look thin and in good shape. Some people may follow the exact workout plan as another and get totally different results. For you, it is a constant trip to the dentist's office that you totally dread. You need to move beyond fairness.

It is our nature to compare because envy is a part of our emotions. Once you achieve a goal, there will always be another one. You may even be the type that no matter what you do, it will never be good enough. *Comparing yourself to others and your past is a losing battle; it only brings anger and resentment.*

Expectations

Why is it so hard to balance my fitness goals and my lifestyle?

Unless you have a paralyzing health problem, there is NO reason not to get some form of exercise; however, you have to be realistic and intelligent while going about it.

If your expectations are too high, you may set yourself up for failure. In some instances, exercise resistance (ER) sets in before you even start.

There has to be a happy medium between goals and lifestyles. Set goals that can fit in with the demands of your life. Manage time better. *Expectations that are too high are self-defeating before you get start.*

John gets a wake up call

After forty-five years of drinking and eating, one or all three of them got to him. The next thing my buddy John knew was he was lying on his back strapped to a heart monitor with a permanent zipper from his belly button to his throat. With a tear in his eye and a cold hand, he said to me, *"If only I had known."*

"This is no time to beat yourself up, John," I told him. "You have been spared. Learn a lesson and move forward." Later on John told me it was his *pride* that got to him.

One out of three of you will break a bone. Half of you are on the verge of obesity and diabetes. A third of you will suffer a heart attack. Half of you will end up in a nursing home. Most of you are not living a life filled with confidence, good sleeping patterns, high energy, or happiness.

Do the math! Numbers do not lie. You either accept the road less traveled or you face the consequences. It is just that simple. This may seem like a scare tactic, but the bottom line is this is reality.

If you think for one second you are exempt, above reproach, or just relying on luck or faith, think again. Your best defense is a good offense. *Denial, Pride* and *Lazy* will always creep in to make you miserable. They are probably already in your life and you do not see them, but you can feel them.

Why now? Resenting the need to exercise is a waste of energy. Never starting because you are afraid of failure is a copout. Striving to exercise to perfection is a bit unrealistic for anyone. Comparing your current condition with how it used to be is a losing battle.

Setting expectations so high that your lifestyle prevents you from accomplishing anything is a "bad attitude ready to happen."

Why now? The bottom line is that you will pay Doctor Joe eventually if you allow any of the excuses to get to you. Exercising and eating right is the best thing you can do for your mind, body, and your heart. It will take work, but the benefits are priceless.

Overview

Let me shoot it to you straight, you are scared. You are fearful of the results of a medical test and the reality your situation. You resent the fact that you have not thought about doing anything until now and you are afraid of not living up to your own expectations. This is fear of looking bad or it being too late to make a difference.

I have three words for you; get over it!

Part 2
AAA Coverage
Acceptance- Attitude-Attraction
(Solving the Problem)

6
Acceptance

Okay, you have acknowledged the fear or fears that are essentially false and delusional thinking. You have also come to grips with the denial you have been in, the pride that has built up, and the sure laziness that you have surrounded yourself with. What is the next step?

Acceptance

This part is huge, so do not just skim over it. Most people have a hard time accepting that they are aging; wrong decisions that they have made; or certain situations from their past.

Accepting and dealing with your circumstance is NOT a sign of weakness, but one of strength. In the beginning, you feel weak, but in the end, you will feel stronger for accepting and dealing with the circumstances. It is funny how that works. Seriously, most people just do not accept their present health issues. They just brush it off and/or ignore it.

Here is a tough question,

"Do you truly feel you deserve to feel better by losing weight?" Think about it.

Self Deserving Prophecy

There is an underlying thought process that you have to acknowledge before you are able to lose weight for good and it is self-deserving. As silly as this may sound, there are those who think they really do not deserve to feel better. They just do not believe they have a right to feel healthier.

Ask yourself, *"Do I deserve to feel better?" "Do I deserve to lose weight?"*

When I first started working out and losing weight, I did not feel in my heart I deserved it. I had such low self-esteem that I believed taking care of me was selfish and unwarranted. Now, I look back and think, *"How sad I must have been and how stupid it was to think that way?"*

Yes, you do deserve to feel better and no, it will not take anything away from anyone else if you do. You may have to believe in yourself a little more.

"Do you really, truly feel you deserve to feel better by losing weight?" Think about it.

7
Attitudes

At this point, it would be much easier to fall back into your old ways. This is human nature. Your head will play games so you just have to find a way to believe.

Believability

I cannot over emphasize what I am about to tell you. Acknowledging the fears is one thing, but dealing with those feelings is entirely another.

I see it every day. People step into my office with good intentions, but deep down they think they are past the point of no return. They have no hope and no believability. Worse than that, some do not even feel they deserve to feel better. Some how, some way, you have to believe you deserve good health before you can achieve it.

Don't Be a Victim

While feeling sorry for yourself at first may make you feel better, in the end your soul will be empty making you feel worse.

At times, life is not fair and things will not always go your way. Feeling like a victim because you cannot or do not lose weight is nothing more than a cop out. The world is not out to get you.

Entitled or Empowered

I grew up in an environment with little to no encouragement. There were rules and you followed them. The farm life required hard work and long hours. The last thing you did was give the impression that you were entitled to anything. You had to earn everything because nothing was given and should not have been expected.

There are basically two types of people in this world; there are givers and there are takers. Each person falls on one side of the fence or the other. Which mind set do you have?

Takers and the Entitled

Takers or the *"Entitled"* have a mindset that the world owes them something. Takers, who are victims by nature, live their lives in fear. At their core, they hate the world because they believe that it has somehow done them wrong. This type of thinking is very draining, fruitless, and, frankly, not positive or productive.

Sooner or later you have to accept the fact that life is not fair; that losing weight takes work; and that losing weight cannot be easily accomplished. The fact is you and I are not entitled to anything. Everything must be earned and it is therefore more appreciated.

Givers or the "Empowered"

Givers or *Empowered* have a different mindset and a much different way of thinking. People that tend to empower people also sway on the side of being thin. Givers do just that because they look to the outside, not the selfish inside. If you want to lose weight, give something away. It sounds corny, but it is the mindset that puts things in motion.

Whether you believe this or not, we attract everything into our lives. If you think your fat, then you are.

8
Laws of Attraction

I do not normally endorse a book within my own, but I believe this is important enough to mention. Like I said, we do not naturally deserve anything, but there are some absolutes in life that come our way.

At this point, you have probably gotten a little used to living in fear, resentment, and all the other negative emotions that come along with it, and there is a reason why.

It is my opinion that we attract most, if not all, things into our lives, which means two things. We can push away bad stuff and then focus on attracting good things. For the sake of this book let us look at moving forward.

Let us also acknowledge that you need to let go of the negative vibes you are sending out. Believe it or not, fear breeds fear. Resentment will follow you like a bad habit. Internal anger will end up making you physically sick. The old saying, "Like attracts like," is very true.

DON'T FORGET TO READ THE LAST CHAPTER!

Part 3
Action Cures Frustration
(Acting on the Problem)

Action cures all frustration!

Greg Ryan

9
Just Move It

This is not a book that outlines the perfect exercise or diet program; however, I want to touch on three key components that guarantee success in any fitness or wellness program when it comes to exercise in particular.

As I said, losing weight is not complicated, but it does take discipline in a few areas. Getting over the fear and feelings that go with it are first important first steps. The second thing is just taking a step.

Action Cures Frustration

An idle mind can get you into trouble. There will always be mental road blocks to break through, so why stay still. I have learned that any type of action toward your goal takes away frustration. What we tend to get frustrated about is not accomplishing the goal so much as it is just trying to. We get mad at ourselves for NOT doing anything when we know we are fully capable. So what is the cure? Just do something.

Exercise

Yes, losing weight takes activity and no, there is no way around it. The problem is that most individuals have the mindset that, "more is better." This is not true. Losing weight through exercise is more about working out smart rather than hard. More is NOT better.

Consistency

No matter how little exercise you decide to undertake, it is important to be consistent with your exercise program. If you walk once a week, then consistently walk once a week.

If you train with weights twice a week, then you should consistently weight training twice a week. Your body will progress and lose weight easier and faster if you are consistent than if you are not. No matter what, plan on being consistent. This goes hand in hand with dieting as well.

Variety

Yes, exercise is boring, especially walking on a treadmill. Be consistent and put some spice in the next workouts.

Most people fail at this and end up quitting their fitness plan because it requires a little pre-planning, which takes brain power.

Adding a little variety into your workouts is not hard and does not require you to change your whole schedule to do so. Take a different path around the park or climb a hill for less time than a flat track. Exercise on a bike instead of a treadmill all the time. Walk in the morning verses the evening hours. What ever it is, never allow your body to get use to the regiment. Again, losing weight is not complicated.

Efficiency

I might not have a PHD in exercise science, but I do have the ability to workout much smarter than most people. The beauty of it is that I do it in half the time that most people exercise in.

Here are a few things I have learned to increase my weight loss success:

1. Set a time limit to your workouts.
2. Work out in the morning.
3. Do a cardio workout before weight training.
4. Exercise the stomach muscles first.

5. Do not take your cell phone when you are work out.
6. Pre-plan your exercises.
7. Set social boundaries during workouts.
8. Use workout time as personal quiet time.
9. Exercise large muscle groups first.
10. Change up your workout plan slightly.

Action cures frustration, but it is not the entire formula. Get rid the fear, act on the frustration, and eat with common sense.

Part 4

Food for Thought, Thoughts for food!
(Eating on the Problem)

10
Planning for Weight Loss

Like exercise, this is not a detailed diet book. Go read *IN OR OUT,* which is my book on food and the behaviors behind them. I would now like to go over some major points about eating for weight loss.

Eating habits are about emotions, pre-planning, and eating for fuel, not for fun. Eating for weight loss is as much about exercising the mind as it is counting the calories.

Busy Minds

Busy minds can induce stress. High stress levels encourage eating foods that taste good, but are incredibly unhealthy.

Busy minds are lazy thinkers. Lazy thinkers are people who go out of their way to get eat for taste rather than for health. You will make better choices when you are faced with fewer pressures in life. If your mind is always running, poor choices are born out of desperation, frustration, and lack of preparation.

Quiet Times

What is quiet time? In today's world, you may find a minute or two to take a breath. Does that really help, though? When is the last time you turned off the radio in your car on the way to work?

When is the last time you turned off your cell phone in the middle of the day? When is the last time you had a cup of coffee from your very *own* coffee machine?

Quiet time means quiet time! If you gave yourself as little as 15 minutes a day for peace and quiet, a lot of your eating habits and food choices would be much easier to handle. They might even disappear. Try it!

Understand, I am not talking about just being by yourself, but I am talking about allowing your mind to rest. Let it take a vacation for 10 minutes. Daydream about something. Read a book. Think of things other than tasks that have to be finished.

Emotions and Eating

You have to eat to live, but why do you eat more food than you need?

This is what you have to figure out. You do not have to be a psychologist. You just need to be aware of the whys behind your eating behaviors. Then you can learn ways to change those ugly habits. Chances are your eating patterns have something to do with an underlying emotion. Emotions do not distinguish between good and bad foods. They just want to be comforted and food is a great blanket!

Lifestyles and Eating

The truth is that you are going to have to change your lifestyle if you want to change your eating habits. This requires some tough choices.

Genetics and Eating

Family history should not be used as a reason not to eat well, but as a platform to do better. If you want to lose weight, you have to consciously monitor your portions of food. Calories add up no matter whether the food is good or bad. Some people by nature can afford to eat more, while others cannot. Be careful because aging lowers metabolism. If you continue to eat the same way as you get older you will naturally gain weight. I never said this was going to be fair.

Blood Sugar Levels and eating

An easy mindset for keeping weight down is to eliminate sugar cravings when possible. I like to establish a daily goal of maintaining my blood sugar by:

- Saying no to heavy meals for lunch or dinner.
- Snacking every four hours.
- Slowing down on white flour foods.
- Eliminating soda pops.
- Slowing down on adding sweets to coffee.

Maintaining even levels of blood sugar cuts your chances of diabetes, obesity, cravings, and binging.

Proper Planning Prevents Poor Performance!

11
The Five P's of Weight Loss

Perspective of eating

If you had the attitude that food was fuel, how would you eat? Would you be more inclined to make better choices? Your attitude toward food is very important! Your self worth, security, and comfort in life does not derive from food. It comes from your heart. Fix your heart and fix the food!

Patterns of eating

It is really important to incorporate a variety of foods in your daily eating program. This keeps your body off guard by preventing it from becoming used to having the same amount of calories. In other words, it lessens the chances of your metabolism slowing down too quickly.

Pushing your buttons

Recognize that advertisers want to push your buttons so you will eat their food. If you plan ahead, you may not have to rely on the fast food industry to eat.

Portions of eating

Learn to push the plate away. Eat with your opposite hand. Put your fork down between shovelfuls. Calories add up, so do what ever you have to do to slow yourself down. Realize you will eat tomorrow!

Planning of eating

This may be the most important behavior of all. If you preplan your week of eating, it will be easier to make better choices. I suggest you go to the grocery store on a scheduled day. This works and I know it! Do you want to lose weight? If so, how bad do you want to lose weight?

Proper planning prevents poor performance!

12
Red Flags

There are some foods that I suggest you watch out for in today's marketplace. By no means are these all of them, but they do rank high on the list of ones to watch out for.

Soda pop

Diet or otherwise, it matters not. Soda pop is a Venus flytrap. High complex carbohydrates and fatty foods stick to soda pop like glue. Soda pop is easily converted into sugar by the body and is non-conducive to your weight loss. If you want to lose a few pounds, you need to lose a few ounces of soda pop. You will be amazed at what happens.

Shelf life and preservatives

The food industry is more interested in the shelf life of food than it is whether the food is healthy for you or not. I always say, "*The more natural, the better.* If at all possible, lower the amount of foods that have additives within your eating plan.

White vs. Wheat

Just as popular as soda are the white flour cravings. White rice, bread, or anything that has an easier time converting into sugar can get you in the end. Try to eliminate or cut down on these types of food as much as possible. Mix them with a glass of wine or soda, and you have a deadly combination.

Non-fat foods

Be careful with non-fat foods. They tend to be full of empty non-nutritious calories. There is nothing wrong with having them, just do not eat them in large quantities. Remember, less is not always better. They may be filling, but they are not very healthy and the calories do add up!

Night time feeding

Heavy carbohydrate meals at night will cause you to put on extra pounds. Watch the high complex carbohydrate foods in the evening hours. Most people do not need high energy foods at night anyway. The more food groups on your plate, the more efficiently the foods will work together to burn fat calories.

Less is more – NOT!

Falling into the trap of eating less in order to avoid gaining weight is a big mistake. It may sound right, but it usually backfires.

The body goes into a protection mode and even slows your metabolism down. The effects of this can be just as bad as eating too much.

Do not mistake fullness for fatness!

All or nothing

Eventually you will crash! Yes, if you decide that one day you are not going to have ice cream again, you will surely fail. Having an "all or nothing" attitude will drive you nuts. You will think about that type of food until you have it. Some unhealthy food, once in a while, is Okay. Just discipline yourself to eat it all of the time. Understand perfectionism can be a psychological disease.

Over view

Diabetes is at an all-time high. Often, when you wait too long between meals, blood sugar levels drop. This is when you may crave foods you normally do not eat.

Control your blood sugar levels daily by watching the types, the amounts, and the times that you eat. Eating right has a lot to do with how you view food, how much you eat, and what you eat.

You need to determine what your eating patterns are. The patterns may be related to lifestyle, emotions, physical concerns, or all the above. Pre-planning meals prevents a lot of the poor decision making. Learn to push yourself away from the table.

Part 5
Just One
(Over Coming the Problem)

PLEASE READ THIS OVER AND OVER!

13
Just One

I have been exercising five days a week for thirty years. The truth is that I hate it. Well, I dislike it a lot. Having said all that, I LOVE the results, but I cannot stand the process. My extended family is extremely over weight. Many of the members have diabetes as well as other illnesses. If I do not keep my weight down, the chances are great that I will end up the same way.

Knowing this does not make the day to day grind any easier. I still have challenges much like everyone else. The fear creeps in daily. My pride is a constant thorn in my side. If I do not monitor myself, I end up, from time to time, swimming in my own denial. What gets me through this? What has kept me going for all these years? I owe credit to just ONE thing.

Every day I get up and I ask God and myself,

"Just for today, please help and let me get through it. It is too difficult to think about tomorrow or the day after that. Just allow me to have the strength, ignore my ego, and push myself off the couch just one more day."

Starting Over Daily

The key to losing weight is facing your fears. Realize that most, if not all, of your fears are delusional thinking on your part. Fear breeds Denial, Pride, and Laziness and when you have one or all three, resentment, anger, envy, strife, and depression sets in.

The only way, and I mean only way, you will survive and be successful losing weight is to **start over every single day.**

Every day I get up thinking it is my first day on the job. What can I do today to make me successful? I do not think about yesterday and what I did not do. I put tomorrow and the things that need to be done out of my mind. All I think about is, just one. Because I know deep down if I do enough *just ones,* then one day I will wake up pounds lighter. I just know it.

What about you? Do you think you can handle just one day at a time? Do you think your weight loss problems stem from fear? If you really think about it, yes they do. Are you mad, frustrated, envious, and/or resentful of your past? If you are honest, yes you are. We cannot help it at times because it is simply human. What we can do is wake up every morning and think, **"Just One."**

Part 6

F

"The only thing to fear is fear itself!"

Franklin D. Roosevelt 1932

14

The Fear Factor

(The Illusion)

Let us put it all in nut shell, simplify it all, and set things in motion.

The reasons you are not losing weight come down to one word, like it or not, and the word is FEAR. FEAR is fueled by two other words, SELF DESERVING and they control the other three words; DENIAL, PRIDE, AND LAZINESS. ALL of these keep you from losing weight.

No matter how you shape it, you have blocked your success with the thoughts in your mind that are simply is not true. You believe them to be true for what ever reason. In the end, maybe they are just easy excuses not to feel better. As crazy as all of these sounds, you know it and I know it, at its core FEAR is our worst enemy.

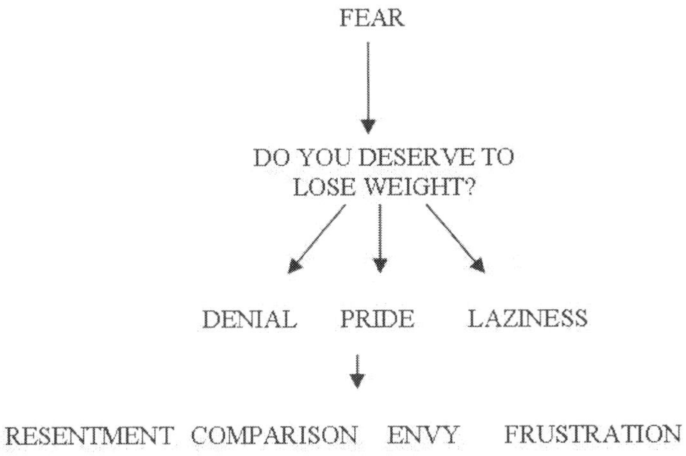
FEAR
DO YOU DESERVE TO LOSE WEIGHT?
DENIAL
PRIDE
LAZINESS
RESENTMENT
COMPARISON
ENVY
FRUSTRATION

Thank You

Thank you for reading **The F Factor!** I wish you all the blessings in the world for this coming year. I trust you have retained something of importance in order to better your health.

As a token of my appreciation, I would like to give you one of my digital books on lowering your body-fat!

Thanks again,
Greg Ryan

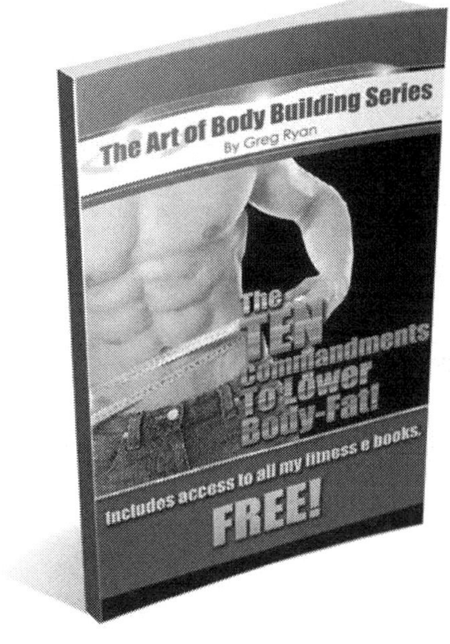
The Art of Body Building Series
By Greg Ryan
The TEN Commandments To Lower Body-Fat!
Includes access to all my fitness e books,
FREE!

Contents

Introduction

Part 1 Mental Body -Fat

I. Balance- Is the Key!

II. Body vs. Mind

Part 2 Physical Body-Fat

III. Body-Fat- What is it and what's the importance of it?

IV. Blood Sugar, Food and Training- The Ultimate Goal!

Part 3 Consumable Body-Fat

V. Binging-Portion Control

VI. Before Noon- Front Loading Carbohydrates

Part 4 Training to Lower Body-Fat

VII. Beliefs to the Core

VIII. Blood Work- Cardiovascular

IX. Body Work- Weight

X. Bonus Material-

Conclusion

Introduction

Too many people focus on the scale, and in the end lose the battle mentally and physically. If you pants are lose, muscles defined and tight, why do you care what the scale registers? Any body can lose or gain weight, but a much less percentage of people keep their body-fat at a respectable level. And very few can maintain it lower than normal for years, I did.

No matter what your age, keeping a lower level of body-fat is vital. If you are of the younger generation then you look better if you are a baby boomer or older a lower fat level is an extremely healthier state of being. This e book outlines just a few ways I have kept my body-fat low for many years. Don't be fooled by the length or lack of gimmicky phrases, its straight for and proven.

There is no magic formula, but there are a few things that will make the process easier.

Part 1
Mental Body-Fat

"Losing body-fat may be just as much mental as physical!"

I
Balance

"You have to constantly juggle your mind and body to lower-body fat!"

Solving the whole body-fat thing can be summed up in one word, *"Balance;"* a much easy word to write than to succeed, I must say.

Balance- *equality between the sums total of the two sides."* In fitness and body-fat there are a few more sides of the equation than just two.

Never Ending Challenge

I was not in a very good mood yesterday and I stated the following to one of my clients, *"If you think for one second that you will work really hard, reach a goal and all will be perfect, you are sorely mistaken and will in the end be very disappointed."*

The same attitude must apply to acquiring an ideal body fat level over time. You must take a life long, day to day approach. Balancing anything in life is usually the biggest challenge any of us will every have. Add the balancing of the ideal workout and eating plan to normal life and it can be doubly as challenging.

The Approach

When I first started workout I had ZERO discipline, faith in myself or confidence that I would or could succeed. Fortunately for some reason I just believed this, *"If I could just get through one day, and one day only at a time then I would worry about tomorrow, well, tomorrow."*

The Attitude

Not to jump ahead but I also learned over time that having a balanced workout, eating and life plan all the time was pretty much impossible.

When one area of the plan is doing well, you have to shift gears to another area. When that one is under control then either the first one or another totally different area of your life and fitness plan needs to be worked on.

My point is this, the goal to lower your body fat is to achieve as close to a balanced plan of all the important things as one possibly can. However, you need to understand that you will never get it perfect, nor if you think you have it, then it will not take long before an area needs more tweaking. You will always be seeking a balanced approach to fitness. The closer you get to it, and the longer you can achieve it, the lower your body-fat will go and stay.

The Area's

There are three main areas I want to focus on in this e book. Each one does not work with out the other. Like a spoke in a wheel with out one the tire will go flat; so goes your body-fat. The three main areas are: Psychology, Nutrition and Physical Training.

Again, allow me to challenge you to take a long term approach, and an attitude that each day will be a constant balancing act of all three areas.

II
Body vs. Mind

"Lowering body-fat takes more faith at times than fitness!"

While a balanced approach is the key, I never said it would be easy. Maintaining the momentum and synergy of everything may come down to more mental than physical. The challenge with the whole subject of body-fat is we can't see it totally. You can look good, but still have less than desirable body-fat levels. The goal is to keep the EGO in check; easier said than done.

Mirrors and Clothes Don't Lie

Man or woman it doesn't matter the mind and EGO is an internal competitor; for woman its vanity, for men it's about being moncho. You can very easily get off base by focusing too much on looks, or bench press numbers, rather than the levels of fat you have.

I've always tried to express to people that at the end of the day, the mirror and clothes don't lie; meaning those two things probably are more accurate of your over all health than a scale. Chances are if your clothes are feeling loser then your body-fat is most likely decreasing; not always though.

What you can't see may kill you

Diabetes is one of the fastest growing diseases today. On some level it seems as though you wake up one morning and you have it; that's really not the case. Developing Diabetes is a process that takes time. Poor eating habits, lack of exercise and genetics all contribute to such a disease. Not being able to see the development of diabetes in our bodies makes us not take it so serious or even increase a state of denial.

The chance's of getting diabetes in your body has been there for some time, but it was not visual so it never crossed your mind. One morning you awake and the doctor says, "Yep, you got it." Diabetes is caused by high levels of body-fat by the way.

You take a similar approach to your body-fat levels, if you can't see it then you assume it's not a problem, or worse yet, not even on the radar screen of life.

Body Fat-Thin is NOT In

Thin is NOT in! When I worked for Kathy Smith in Los Angeles, California I managed about fifty employees; ten of them were aerobic instructors. Out of the ten half weighed an average of 115 pounds. The shocking thing was come to find out through a club testing day most of them were clinically considered obese. What? How can that be? By looking at them you would draw the conclusion that they were in great shape; and to the public eye they were.

Thin is NOT In

The tests discovered that over thirty percent of their total body weight was in the form of fat, medically, making them fit into the obese category; totally shocking to the naked eye. So be very careful not to distort the idea that thinness equals healthiness.

In short for the instructors, to high heart rate over time ate away at muscle tissue, combined with poor eating habits eventually made their ratio of muscle to overall body weight out of balance.

Contrast this with some football players who are big and bulky and the same thing occurs, too much weight and a decrease in muscle can make you obese with out looking like it.

Part 2
Physical Body-Fat

"Understanding what body-fat is and the importance of lowering it is half the battle!"

III
Body-Fat

"Getting muscular or losing weight is one thing, lowering your body-fat is another story!"

What is Body-Fat?

Body fat is a compound comprised of glycerol -- a substance formed in fatty acids -- and fatty acids which is required as a concentrated energy source for our muscles. Fat is a storage substance for the body's extra calories and it fills fat cells (adipose tissue) that help insulate the body. When the body has used up the calories from carbohydrates it begins to depend on the calories from fat.

How can I determine body fat percentage?

There are several ways to find out your body fat percentage. Unfortunately, the more accurate the method, the more of a hassle and/or expensive it tends to be.

DEXA scan – full body X-ray scan of the same type used for bone density. Very accurate.

Hydrostatic Weighing - Weighing under water (completely submerged, with all air blown out of lungs) - Very accurate when done professionally.

Skin-fold calipers ("pinch test") - Simple, but needs to be done by someone who is trained, and you can't do it on yourself. Wide variations in accuracy for people without training.

Bioelectrical Impedance (BIA) - These are scales and hand-held devises that run low-level (and painless) electrical current through you. They can be accurate, although the accuracy varies according to the specific device (do your research) and how it is used. Best results are obtained first thing in the morning with no alcohol consumed for 2 days prior, and no exercise the night before.

Navy tape measure method - This is a formula based on several body measurements taken with a tape measure. It can be quite accurate (it is used by the military), but it does depend upon your ability to accurately measure. Using centimeters rather than inches is the best, but using inches within ¼ of an inch works. To be sure, measure yourself 3 times and take the average.

What's the difference between Body Fat Percentage and BMI?

BMI (body mass index) is a formula based on height and weight. It was developed because in the general population, it is correlated with body fat. However, there are quite a few groups of people for whom BMI is not as accurate -- short women and muscular people, to name two.

BMI also varies according to some ethnic groups. Also, for people who are interested in changing their body composition and not just their weight, knowing body fat percentage is an improvement over BMI. For example, if you are exercising to build muscle (a good goal), knowing your body fat percentage is a good idea.

Also, when losing weight, you want to preserve as much lean body mass as possible. (Low-carb diets generally produce better results than high carb ones for this purpose.)

If you want to lose or gain weight, you need to be able to measure the state your body is in now and then monitor the changes as you add or subtract calories from your diet. One way to do this is to calculate and monitor your Body Mass Index (BMI).

Since a typical scale only measures your total weight, it helps to have more information to determine if that weight is healthy or unhealthy. A person who is six feet tall and weighs 198 pounds is probably going to have a smaller amount of body fat than a person who is five feet tall and 198 pounds.

The BMI combines your weight and your height into a score that helps you determine if you are underweight, at a healthy weight, overweight, or obese.

BMI is calculated with the following formula:

weight (lb) / [height (in)]^2 x 703

or in metric:

weight (kg) / [height (m)]^2

What Your BMI Means

You can compare your BMI to this table to help you determine whether you're at a healthy weight.

- Underweight = less than 18.5
- Normal weight = 18.5-24.9
- Overweight = 25-29.9
- Obese = 30 or greater

If you are planning to lose or gain weight, you can use your BMI to monitor your progress. It's important to know that your BMI is not the same as your body fat percentage, which is a different number and doesn't correspond to these charts.

People who have a BMI in the overweight or obese ranges may have a higher risk of cardiovascular disease, diabetes, arthritis, and some forms of cancer. However, it's important to see your health care provider, who can take other lifestyle and risk factors into consideration.

The BMI isn't perfect because it's an indirect measurement of fat, and really doesn't differentiate pounds of fat from pounds of muscle and bone. So it doesn't work well for very muscular people or for people who have lost a lot of muscle mass.

For example, an elite athlete with a very small amount of body fat will still have a high BMI, and an elderly person may have a lower BMI because they have less muscle mass. In these cases, a better method of measurement is the body fat percentage.

By the Numbers

If you are a numbers person here are ones to shoot for when trying to lower your body fat.

Age	Under fat	Healthy Range	Overweight	Obe
20-40 yrs	Under 21%	21-33%	33-39%	Ove
41-60 yrs	Under 23%	23-35%	35-40%	Ove
61-79 yrs	Under 24%	24-36%	36-42%	Ove

Men

Age	Under fat	Healthy Range	Overweight	Obe
20-40 yrs	Under 8%	8-19%	19-25%	Ove
41-60 yrs	Under 11%	11-22%	22-27%	Ove
61-79 yrs	Under 13%	13-25%	25-30%	Ove

Above Average Below Grade

Unfortunately most of you are above the average, and in the body-fat category anything above is not good. So what grade will you give yourself?

There are many things that contribute to higher body-fat but in this book we will only concentrate on a few of the things that will give you more bang for the buck. For me there a few major things that I concentrated on daily that helped me keep my body-fat low for years.

IV
Blood Sugar

"Blood Sugar, Food and Training- The Ultimate Goal!"

For the last twenty five years or so I have had one daily goal. I found by achieving this goal each day, my body-fat would stay at a lower level. I understood that if I monitored and regulated my blood sugar levels through good nutritional habits, and a balanced exercise program the rest would kind of fall into place.

What is Blood Sugar?

In short, blood **sugar** concentration or blood glucose level **is** the amount of glucose (**sugar**) present in the blood.

Blood sugar, also known as blood glucose, is the body's fuel that feeds the brain, nervous system, and tissues. A healthy body makes glucose not only from ingested carbohydrates, but also from proteins and fats, and would not be able to function without it.

Maintaining a balanced blood glucose level is essential to a body's everyday performance.

Glucose is absorbed directly into the bloodstream from the intestine and results in a rapid increase in the blood glucose level. The pancreas releases insulin, a natural hormone, to prevent blood glucose levels from excessively elevating, and aids in the moving of glucose into the cells. Glucose is then carried to each cell, providing them with the energy needed to carry out its specific function.

Healthy blood glucose levels are considered to be in the 70-120 range. One high or low reading does not always indicate a problem, but the glucose level should be monitored for 10-14 days. There are several different tests that can be administered to determine whether an individual has a problem maintaining a normal glucose level such as: a fasting blood sugar test, an oral glucose test, or a random blood sugar test. Blood glucose levels that remain either too high or too low over time may cause damage to the eyes, kidneys, nerves and blood vessels.

Hypoglycemia

Hypoglycaemia is a condition caused by low blood sugar levels in the body, can be extremely debilitating if not controlled properly. Symptoms include shaking, irritability, confusion, strange behaviour and even loss of consciousness. These symptoms can be corrected by ingesting a form of a sugar such as a hard candy, a sugar pill, or a sweet drink. Ingesting one or more of these forms of sugar quickly raises the body's blood sugar level and has an almost immediate effect.

Hyperglycemia

Hyperglycemia occurs when the blood glucose levels in the body are higher than normal. Symptoms of this condition include: excessive thirst, frequent urination, tiredness, weakness and lethargy. If the levels become excessively high, a person can become dehydrated and comatose.

A Side Note

Diabetes occurs when the pancreas either produces little or no insulin, or the cells do not respond appropriately to the insulin produced. There are three main types of diabetes: Type 1, Type 2, and Gestational Diabetes. Type 1 diabetes occurs when the body's immune system attacks insulin producing cells in the pancreas destroying them and causing the pancreas to produce little or no insulin. Type 2 diabetes is the most common and is associated with age, obesity, and genetics. Gestational diabetes develops only during pregnancy, but means an increase in the chance of the woman developing Type 2 diabetes in the future. All types of diabetes are serious and need to be monitored regularly.

Insulin Resistance

What is insulin resistance?

Insulin resistance is a condition in which the body produces insulin but does not use it properly. Insulin, a hormone made by the pancreas, helps the body use glucose for energy. Glucose is a form of sugar that is the body's main source of energy.

The body's digestive system breaks food down into glucose, which then travels in the bloodstream to cells throughout the body. Glucose in the blood is called blood glucose, also known as blood sugar. As the blood glucose level rises after a meal, the pancreas releases insulin to help cells take in and use the glucose.

When people are insulin resistant, their muscle, fat, and liver cells do not respond properly to insulin. As a result, their bodies need more insulin to help glucose enter cells. The pancreas tries to keep up with this increased demand for insulin by producing more.

Eventually, the pancreas fails to keep up with the body's need for insulin. Excess glucose builds up in the bloodstream, setting the stage for diabetes. Many people with insulin resistance have high levels of both glucose and insulin circulating in their blood at the same time.

Insulin resistance increases the chance of developing type 2 diabetes and heart disease. Learning about insulin resistance is the first step toward making lifestyle changes that can help prevent diabetes and other health problems.

What causes insulin resistance?

Scientists have identified specific genes that make people more likely to develop insulin resistance and diabetes. Excess weight and lack of physical activity also contribute to insulin resistance.

Many people with insulin resistance and high blood glucose have other conditions that increase the risk of developing type 2 diabetes and damage to the heart and blood vessels, also called cardiovascular disease.

These conditions include having excess weight around the waist, high blood pressure, and abnormal levels of cholesterol and triglycerides in the blood. Having several of these problems is called metabolic syndrome or insulin resistance syndrome, formerly called syndrome X.

Roller (coaster)

A good indicator (or one for me) that my blood sugar levels were off during the day was my tiredness around mid morning and afternoon.

If you look at roller coasters you will basically find two kinds; hilly ones and those that just go straight up and down. Or maybe we could visualize a one hump camel or a two humped one. Either way, the goals is to not have too many humps (ups and downs) in your blood sugar levels through out the day.

Two Humped Camels

When your blood sugar levels or energy levels go up and down like a two humped camel you DO NOT burn body-fat. Chances are you will probably do the opposite of what you should do. (See the nutritional chapter)

The Five Hour Energy Craze

Each year American's consume about eight hundred million dollars of the product called, "Five Hour Energy Drink."

Why, because, most people are tired either mid morning or mid afternoon? The drink apparently revives you long enough (five hours) to get through the rest of your day. All it is is caffeine and mineral water. The company is basically making boat loads of money off of people's LAZINESS.

I really believe that people's biggest problem of obesity and high body-fat levels is due to poor regulation of their blood sugars caused by lack of exercise and poor eating habits.

Blood Sugar Regulation

Blood sugar levels are regulated by negative feedback in order to keep the body in homeostasis.
The levels of glucose in the blood are monitored by the cells in the pancreas's Islets of Langerhans. If the blood glucose level falls to dangerous levels (as in very heavy exercise or lack of food for extended periods), the Alpha cells of the pancreas release glucagon, a hormone whose effects on liver cells act to increase blood glucose levels.

They convert glycogen into glucose (this process is called glycogenolysis). The glucose is released into the bloodstream, increasing blood sugar levels.

While far as I know I am not diabetic or even pre-diabetic, however for me the whole ball of wax came down to, ***"HOW do I control and regulate my blood sugar levels every single day?"*** It came down to two categories; eating and exercising smart.

Here are a few ways I regulated by blood sugar levels:

Eat often
Never skip breakfast
Don't eat past 8 at night
No white flour at noon or evening meals
Protein snacks between meals
Workout in the morning

Part 3
Consumable Body-Fat

"Balance the diet and solve your body-fat issue, half way!"

V
Binging- Portion Control

"Control the roller coaster and cure the body-fat!"

Call it any thing you want, but eating to much food in too little time in my mind is binging; and binging cause blood sugar problems which in the long run raises body-fat levels.

If you really want to know how much you are eating, just calculate all the calories you consume in a day, or in each meal at the very least. I would be willing to bet you would be surprised and even shocked at the amount of calories consumed or inhaled.

You always hear about snacking and eating smaller meals through out the day, why? By nature we eat more when we eat less often.

One feeds on the other

We talked about blood sugar levels and the important of keeping them even through out the day.

But it also must be noted how low blood sugar levels promote bigger portion sizes, in turn larger portion sizes spike blood sugar levels and then they crash. Each one feeds on the other building up so much momentum that in some cases if you don't exercise you run the risk of becoming pre-diabetic or worse full blown diabetes.

VI
Before Noon
"Early bird gets the energy"

If I have any secrets to keeping my body fat lower than most here's one of them; I front load my carbohydrates daily.

Carbohydrate FRONT Loading

What the heck do you mean Front loading your carbohydrates?

Let's look at the habits of most people. One reason so many people have gotten fatter over the years is because of convenience, laziness and lack of planning their foods. What food group is the easiest to get and fix? Yes, carbohydrates. And when do people eat the majority of those carbohydrates, at night, right? What do carbohydrates supply to the body? Yes, energy. When do we need the most energy, at night or in the morning? So, what's wrong with this picture then?

Eating good food can still make you fat

In the early nineties a study came out on how good pasta was for you, so what did people do? They ate more pasta. American's are almost twenty percent fatter today than back then. How can that be, pasta was suppose to be good for you? It is, however, consumed at night followed by a night on your back, converts into glucose and over time, fat.

Front Loading

You hear of carbohydrate loading in sports so I guess you could say that I carbohydrates loaded to keep my body-fat low. Well a better and more accurate way of saying it is, I FRONT loaded my carbohydrate intake. In other words, if I want to keep my body-fat lower I will eat the majority of my carbohydrates, more importantly the complex carbs prior to the two o'clock hour.

Part 4
Training to Lower Body-Fat

"Physical exercise is like a tool of a sculpture, if used just enough, art is created!"

VII
Beliefs from the Core

"Having a little faith may be the most important action to lower body-fat!"

The core muscle groups may be the most functional and important muscle groups in your body. They also may be the most neglected out of them all as well.

Your Belief System

One thing I learned early on in my body building career was that you have to have a strong belief in working out your core muscles. It's very easy to make any excuse NOT to exercise the core muscles.

The other thing is, they HURT. Doing core muscle group exercises are painful, so you have to believe in what you are doing at the time, a little faith goes along ways.

Faith

Having faith in something you can't see is challenging to say the least. Just looking at your body in the mirror is no accurate way of measuring body-fat. You can't even muster a good guess by a visual.

VIII
Blood Work

In the beginning chapter of this book we discussed the importance of being balanced. When it comes to physical training to lower your body-fat it's a dicey path. It really is a balancing act of good food, sleep, a stress free attitude, cardiovascular and strength training. The goal is to rid the body of fat while at the same time continue to develop lean muscle tissue.

Blood Flow- Cardiovascular Training

Just walking, biking, crossfit or step class does not cut it when it comes to losing weight and body-fat. I can not remember the last I went into a gym and saw a member check their heart rate zone.

Target Heart Rate Zone

There is no way you will get to your ideal body-fat weight unless you hit your target heart rate zone every time you perform cardiovascular training.

Don't go over or under, you have to hit the target. If you go over you burn valuable muscle, under and weight stays on. Memorize this formula;

220-age x 60-85% = Target Heart Rate (THR)

Cardiovascular Training Protocol

Like I said, I never see people take their heart rates, machine or by hand. So here is the protocol you should follow to lower the fat levels efficiently:

1. First and fore most calculate your heart rate numbers. You only have to do this once and memorize the zone and divide by six.
2. No matter what cardiovascular piece of equipment you use by the seven minute mark of your workout you should and must be in your zone. Most people are not in there until twelve to fifteen minutes in.
3. Maintain this zone for a minimum of twenty minutes and a maximum of forty minutes.
4. Don't just get off of the equipment at the end, slow the pace down gradually; this is the cool-down

period. Cardiac arrest may occur if you don't cool down properly.

Cannibalism

Cannibals eat their own. If you exercise with your heart rate to high your muscles eat their own.

The average weight of my aerobic instructors in LA was around 115 pounds. After a surprise body-fat test, over half were clinically obese. How is that possible? Cannibalism!

Day after day they failed to monitor their heart rates, thus they were too high. Day after day their bodies were not being fueled properly for their training regiment. With the combination of the two, their body's recuperation process could not keep up with the demand they had been putting on themselves. Over time, precious muscle tissue was being eaten away like hungry, desperate pack man. Eventually, the percentage of body-fat to their over all weight was close or over thirty percent, clinically obese numbers. Ouch!

More is not better either!

Don't make the mistake of trying to put logic with exercise, your dealing with a human body that in the end will not be able to totally manipulate. Those aerobic instructors for some reason thought that the more they did, the higher they kept their heart rates the less they would weight and lower the body-fat. Unfortunately, all that did was hurt their health not help it.

Cycle Intensity Levels

Adaptation is a word you will hear me say frequently. I truly believe the body is smart and has a good memory. This will take some pre-planning on your part, however, maybe one of the smartest and most effective techniques I have used in keeping my body-fat low over the years.

In other words, never do the same identical cardiovascular workout three times in a row. This can be accomplished by changing length of workouts, elevations or intensity levels, time during the day or even locations.

IX
Body Work

Cardiovascular is aerobic and weight training is anaerobic, we all know this, however, there is one little thing I have discovered over the years when it comes to weight training and body-fat.

We are all taught as well as you have learned in this book that a combination of food, cardiovascular and now weight training aids in lowering body-fat. Now let's dissect this theory a little bit more in detail as it pertains to weight training and body-fat.

Flipping the Switch

I truly believe that you can keep your body-fat lower over time more so than even most people imagine as it pertains to weights. Not so much the exercises, but the technique in which you go through the workouts. Over the years I learned to flip a switch right before I walked into the gym.

Time Lines

The first thing I did was, decide to put a time limit to my weight training workouts.
Whether I was done with my body-parts or not I would walk out of the gym. Walking out once or twice cured me of messing around.

The Art of Flow

I have been complimented time and time again for how artful my workouts look. From afar there seems to be a sense of methodical flow from rep to set, exercise to machine; an effortless motion. Like I mentioned, flipping the mental switch and times lines cut my time down between sets and exercises and in the long run by doing this my body-fat stayed lower.

Call it, flow, intensity, focus what ever you want to, all I know is, body-fat stayed off, I had more fun and received more results in a shorter period of time.

X
Bonus

Variety

I am convinced that our bodies get bored with what we do physically, adapt and plateau in getting results. Mentally we get stale and that translates into physical stagnation. Then what do you do? You quit.

Pre Planning

Putting variety into your workouts and eating habits takes a little thinking ahead; this is why most don't do it, its too much work. However, pre-planning your workouts and eating accomplishes two things, takes a lot of wasted energy and time out of your life and builds confidence, which in turn creates momentum.

Workout Variety

Our bodies start getting use to repetitive actions with in our workouts around six to eight weeks into a workout plan.

I really can not explain it, but the body assumes you are going to do the same exercise, weight and order of those exercises after a certain time. When this happens the body plateaus and in some cases the body fat goes up, because the heart rate stays at a lower rate through out the workout.

Food Variety

Maybe it's the typical number of calories, I'm not sure but just as with a typical workout for you the body gets use to the same old foods you eat as well. If you have oatmeal and wheat toast every morning for breakfast even though the food types are good for you the calorie amount stays the same. Over time the body gets use to that amount of calories and again, the metabolism slows down.

Conclusion

For overall health stand point, there is nothing more valuable than keeping your body-fat in check. If you are concerned about appearance, a body never looks better than lean and mean. Achieving such a goal is not as hard as *keeping* ones body-fat lower; it really does take a *balanced* approach.

In my opinion, it's easy to put on muscle or lose weight, but it's much more difficult to do both at the same time; its quality not quantity. Quality muscle and low body mass takes a juggling act on a consistent basis and in the end it maybe more of a *mind* game than anything.

In order to over come something you have to understand what it is and why its there. Body-fat is not Body Mass. Body-fat is not necessarily pounds read on a scale either.

Remember to keep the first things first, and always focus on *blood sugar.* If you regulate your blood sugar the body-fat has to stay low. I realize life is hectic these days, however some way some how you have to *pre plan*, set goals and be proactive verses reactive. If you don't, you will constantly eat more than you should, throwing your metabolism into a free fall.

Body-fat tends to come off easier when the metabolism stays constant through out the day not the evening so watch those high energy foods late at night. You have to realize that it's not all about exercise, it's about food too. But when you do exercise more is NOT better. Be smart, efficient and precise. Monitor your efforts, structure with variety works best for me. You do all this one day you will awake and guess what, the switch is flipped and the body-fat has gone.

Its not rocket science, but it will take work. And I know you've heard this a lot, but seriously, if I've done this you can too; one goal, one day, one meal, one workout, one percent body-fat at a time.

Good Luck!

Greg Ryan

I have a wealth of FREE information on weight loss, fitness, nutrition and bodybuilding.

Website: www.resolutions.bz
Email: greg@resolutions.bz

FREE Fitness Advice

Blogs:

www.resolutionsblog.com
www.reso-care.com
www.gregryanfitness.com

Check out my entire book collection at